What Every Parent Should Know About Autism

Understanding How to Care for an Autistic Child

by

SHEENA ELLY

Legal & Disclaimer

The information contained in this book and its contents is not designed to replace or take the place of any form of medical or professional advice; and is not meant to replace the need for independent medical, financial, legal or other professional advice or services, as may be required. The content and information in this book has been provided for educational and entertainment purposes only.

The content and information contained in this book has been compiled from sources deemed reliable, and it is accurate to the best of the Author's knowledge, information and belief. However, the Author cannot guarantee its accuracy and validity and cannot be held liable for any errors and/or omissions. Further, changes are periodically made to this book as and when needed. Where appropriate and/or necessary, you must consult a professional (including but not limited to your doctor, attorney, financial advisor or such other professional advisor) before using any of the suggested remedies, techniques, or information in this book.

Upon using the contents and information contained in this book, you agree to hold harmless the Author from and against any damages, costs, and expenses, including any legal fees potentially resulting from the application of any of the information provided by this book. This disclaimer applies to any loss, damages or injury caused by the use and application, whether directly or indirectly, of any advice or information presented, whether for breach of contract, tort, negligence, personal injury, criminal intent, or under any other cause of action.

You agree to accept all risks of using the information presented inside this book.

You agree that by continuing to read this book, where appropriate and/or necessary, you shall consult a professional (including but not limited to your doctor, attorney, or financial advisor or such other advisor as needed) before using any of the suggested remedies, techniques, or information in this book.

Table of Contents   Page

Introduction

Autism is known as a disorder of the neural development of a person, which is routinely defined by both impeded communication and social interaction. It is also characterized by behavior that is both repetitive as well as restrictive. All of these signs of autism can be observed in people when they are still very young, usually before the age of 3. This disorder has a reputation for impacting how the brain processes information through changing how both nerve cells as well as their synapses associate and get organized. Because of the aforementioned problems that stem from autism, it is a disorder that clearly creates a lot of lifestyle dilemmas for the person who has to endure this disorder.

For one, the social development of a person is highly impacted by autism in a negative way. People with autism have to endure social impediments and so frequently fail to have the normal social intuitions about all the other people they come across. This lack of proper social development is apparent already from early childhood onwards. For example, it starts with autism experiencing infants already showing less attention to stimulus in their environment, reacting less often to their own name than their peers and smiling less frequently than their normal peers, too.

As adults, people with autism will have to deal more frequently with more intense loneliness than their peers who do not have autism. It comes as no surprise, then, that people with autism will also have a lifestyle where they will have fewer friendships than their non-autistic peers, primarily since it is challenging for them to make and keep friends. For these people, it is the quality of their friendships and not the number of their friends that establishes the extent of their loneliness. Friendships that are functional, like ones that result in invites to parties, might have an even more profound effect on their lifestyle.

What this book covers

Communication is another aspect of lifestyle that is harshly hampered by autism. In fact, up to 50 percent of all autism patients actually come short of developing satisfactory natural speech to satisfy their everyday communication requirements! Just imagine how awfully and how brutally this will affect such a person's lifestyle. Interestingly, though, persons who speak with autism patients initially assume that said autistic folks can understand more than they really can.

The repetitive behavior that is seen in those who have autism also negatively impacts their lifestyle. For instance, repetitive behavior can include things such as self-injury (repeated head banging or picking at skin), a ritualistic behavior that involves doing the same thing each day and compulsive behavior that involves a rigid adherence to rules.

Clearly, people with autism display a lot of behavioral patterns that normal people would derogate as "weird." as such, this leads to autistic people having a lot more difficulty in dealing with people and being social. As a result, the impact of autism on the lifestyle of an autistic person is very negative and forces her to deal with a lot of challenges.

Chapter 1 Recognizing Your Child's Uniqueness

The key to understanding the condition of your child with autism is being able to recognize how his mind and body works.

Defining Autism

To put it simply, autism is a disorder affecting the brain and behavioral functions of your child. Because of his condition, your child experiences difficulties in his social interactions, engages in rigid actions that he tends to do over and over again, and suffers from stunted development of his communication and language skills.

A wide range of levels of impairment, skills, and symptoms are involved in this condition, and these are manifested in different ways in different children with autism. Some may be handicapped and struggle to live a normal life, while others may need continuous care from a professional treatment program.

Autism Signs

Communication troubles. Difficulty in communicating with others is one of the symptoms of autism. Your child tends to have problems grasping the thoughts and feelings of other people, which make it difficult for him to express himself, whether verbally or through body language (facial expressions, gestures, and touch).

Hypersensitivity. Your child can be particularly sensitive. This causes him to be troubled and/or pained by regular sights, smells, sounds, and touches.

Repetitive movements. It is not unusual for your child with autism to have stereotyped body movements (including hand flapping, pacing, and rocking), which he will do repetitively.

Odd reactions. On the one hand, your child may form an unusual attachment to certain objects. On the other hand, it would seem at times that your child does not notice the objects, people, and even the activities going on in his environment. He tends to resist any change he encounters in his routines, act awkwardly around other people, and act in aggressive ways that can cause him to injure himself.

Seizures. Your child may develop seizures, which may or may not occur until he reaches the adolescent stage.

Irregular development of skills. To a certain degree, a number of children with autism may have cognitive impairment. Unlike what you would typically observe in other children, where they may experience delays in all development areas, your child may show development problems in some areas only (of which the more obvious are his communication and socialization skills).

What is surprising is that these developmental delays in skills are seemingly compensated by his excellent abilities in other areas, like facts memorization, drawing, math problems solving, or music creation. This is why your child may get higher test scores in intelligence tests that are of the non-verbal type.

Onset Of Symptoms

The initial three years of your child's life is the typical stage in which autism symptoms occur, although there are cases wherein a child may show signs of autism from birth. Some children with autism show normal signs of development in the beginning, and then suddenly exhibit symptoms of autism once they turn 1 ½ years to 3 years old.

Scope of Autism

Role of environment. There have been cases in which the demands of a person's environment cannot be met by his capabilities, and this is what causes him to suddenly experience communication problems and show other autism signs.

Commonness in males. Boys have been found to be four times as likely to have autism as girls.

Pervasiveness across boundaries. Autism cuts across boundaries (social status, race, or ethnicity), and its likelihood of affecting a child is not dependent on his parents' lifestyle, educational attainment, or income.

Autism's Roots

Genetics. Autism has been found to run in families, which has prompted a great number of researchers to believe that there are particular gene pools that increase a child's likelihood to have autism.

Risk factors. There are risk factors, however, that can affect your child's potential of having the disorder: obesity and diabetes due to pregnancy (or other maternal metabolic conditions), as well as the use of alcohol and anti-seizure drugs while pregnant. Untreated PKU (phenylketonuria) and rubella (German measles) have also been linked to autism.

Brain abnormality. The reason that autism occurs is still unclear up to this day. What is suggested by studies is that there are certain areas in the brain (language processing and sensory input interpretation) that may play roles in a child's cognitive impairment.

Parent's advanced age. A mother who gets pregnant and gives birth at an advanced age seems to have increased risk of having a child with autism.

Mother's chemical exposure. Being exposed to certain chemicals

Chapter 2 Teaching Your Structure Dependent Child

Effectively teaching your child with autism can be a challenging task, especially when you have to consider his need for structure. But with the help of these tips, helping your child learn can actually be both engaging and rewarding.

Significance Of Structure

When you give your child the gift of learning with structure, you are also helping reduce his feelings of stress, anxiety, and confusion, and this makes him less likely to behave in difficult or problematic ways. Teaching your child with structure in mind is also one way of capitalizing on his strengths – predictability, repetitiveness, routine, organization, and the need for finality. Structure may even help your child become more independent.

Providing Structure To Your Child's Learning Process

The following are helpful tips on teaching your structure dependent child:

Be predictable with your child's schedule. It helps to design a predictable learning schedule for your child. Many children with autism find it beneficial when they are taught on a schedule that they can rely on to take place without any changes. A predictable learning schedule helps your child feel more secure because he knows what will happen every day.

TRY: Placing an analog or a digital clock that is clearly visible on a wall in your house. You can also put up pictures of your child's daily activities along with the specific times in which they occur. You may then refer to the clock and the pictures as you cue your child on his activities.

Keep your child's lessons short and simple. Your language should be concrete and simple at all times. It helps to use fewer words when getting a particular point across, instead of going for lengthy verbal instructions. Your child can also have a difficulty in remembering sequences, which is why instructions that consist of no more than three steps are ideal.

TRY: Instead of looking out the window and then vaguely telling your child that "the air outside feels so cool," say "Put your pen down, stand up, and go outside with me." Once your child is able to read, make sure to write down directions to help him follow through the steps.

Do repetitions of instructions without modifications. It always helps to ensure that your child listens to what you say to him and that he understands them. There are many children with autism who have been observed to look at their parent or teacher intently, without truly absorbing whatever is being said or taking place. This is why you will need to repeat everything you say, especially if you are not sure that your child has understood you.

TRY: Give your child more time in processing all the information that he gets from you. It also helps to make sure that when you repeat your instruction to your child, you should say the instruction in the same way you did the first time. Modifying the steps ever so slightly will only burden your child with the task of having to process the new information.

Set a defined learning area. It will help your child's need for structure if the learning area is clearly defined. This addresses his need for organization and predictability, which is hard to accomplish when the learning area is chaotic or is held in different settings.

TRY: Define the different areas of your child's learning area by constructing separate stations for his books, crafts, and toys. You can also place physical markers on the floor to clearly indicate your child's play and reading area, among other things.

Be direct. It helps to never fail to address your child by his name. This will help him understand that you are talking to him, especially if there happens to be other people around. Make sure that you inject a positive note in your instruction.

TRY: Don't rely on your tone of voice to make him come to you after you vaguely say "come here." You have to call him by his name. You should also say "slow down" instead of "stop running" to keep things on the positive side.

Don't be in a hurry. Transitions are difficult to deal with for your structure dependent child, which is why preparatory commands are a must when teaching him. Make sure that you phrase your commands carefully to effectively cue you're your child in on what is going to happen next.

TRY: Say to your child "In ten minutes we will finish reading the book and talk about it."

Recognize your child's learning framework. Identify the learning framework that your child has created for himself. He may use certain objects, exhibit particular behaviors, or engaging in some rituals that enable him to learn or memorize things. Your child may be more comfortable learning the alphabet while he walks, or feel more at ease reading aloud while holding his favorite blanket.

Show your child what he needs to do exactly. It helps to let your child know how you want something to get finished. This will also help him figure out when he needs to go on to the next task. Show your child a photo of a finished activity or product you would like him to get started on. For example, let him see a picture of what a clean room looks like if you want him to tidy up his room.

Chapter 3 Helping Your Visual Thinking Child Learn

As a child who has autism, our child is a natural visual thinker. His first language most likely consists of pictures, and his second language involves words. You could say that his thoughts run through his mind like a series of videos.

Harnessing Your Child's Visual Thoughts

Nouns. Children with autism learn best when they can form in their minds a picture of a certain word, which is why the easiest words for them to learn are nouns. It will help a lot if you show your child the movements associated with the words "up" and "down" – say "up" as you demonstrate his toy airplane taking off from a table. You could also try attaching the word "down" to the toy airplane when you make it land on the table.

Numbers. Teaching number concepts to your child becomes easier when you use visual methods that are concrete, such as a math toy that consists of blocks of varying lengths and colors (each of the numbers one to ten is assigned its own length and color). Your child will be able to learn about numbers, especially addition and subtraction, by playing with this math toy.

Meanwhile, you can help your child learn about fractions by cutting up an apple-shaped wood into four pieces and a pear-shaped wood into two pieces. Working with these wooden pieces will let him learn about halves and quarters.

Phonics. Your child may be one of those kids with autism who learns to read more easily when using phonics, in which you make him sound out the words he learns. If your child happens to engage in plenty of echolalia, you will find that using picture books and flash cards are a big help when it comes to reading. This will help your child associate each word with a particular picture, especially if the word is printed on the page or card's side that the picture can be found.

Captions. Processing the spoken words he hears can also be difficult for your child to do, which is the reason it helps to make use of those closed captions usually used on TV. Your child can easily learn new words, whether or not he already knows how to read. He will readily associate the spoken words he hears with the printed words he sees on the television. If a particular TV show is your child's favorite, you can make a record of that show and then have him watch it as part of your reading activity.

Managing Your Child's Visual Challenges

Flicker. Problems with visual processing are common in children with autism. This condition makes them more sensitive to the appearance of flicker in certain computer monitors. Help reduce your child's visual difficulties by letting him use a computer with a flat-panel display or a laptop computer, which tends to flicker less.

Escalators. Visual processing troubles are also the most likely reason that a number of adults and kids are afraid of using escalators. Your child may have a fear of getting on an escalator since it is hard for him to pinpoint the perfect time for him to get on or get off.

Fluorescent lights. Your child may also show low tolerance for the glare given off by fluorescent lights. You can buy prescription colored glasses to help your child get around this particular issue.

Black print. It is common in children with autism to have problems with visual processing, leading them to find it less difficult to read a low-contrast reading material. Choose books that use black characters printed on colored pages, such as gray, tan, light blue, or light green. The one color to avoid is bright yellow, since it can hurt your child's eyes (although this can be remedied if he uses prescription colored glasses).

Chapter 4 Being More In Sync With Your Child

Out Of Sync Senses

Having autism causes your child to have his senses out of sync. Ordinary things that other children and adults take for granted can make him feel excruciating pain, such as touches, sounds, sights, and smells that are hardly noticeable. All of these make your child feel that he is living in a hostile environment, causing him to withdraw or act belligerent, when in fact these things are merely his defense mechanisms.

Storm of sounds. Your child's sense of hearing can be so acute that the loud sounds coming from the school bell cause his ears to feel as though a nerve was hit by a dentist while drilling. Because your child's ears are easily hurt by loud sounds, it is important that you take measures to protect them. In school, the most problematic sources of hurtful sounds are chairs make as they scrape on the floor, buzzers on the gym's score board, PA systems, and school bells.

You might be able to find a way to have the buzzers or school bells muffled slightly (stuffing duct tape or tissues into them can work) so that your child will be able to tolerate the sounds coming from them. You might arrange for chairs to not make scraping sounds by having carpet installed or having slit tennis balls placed at the bottom of the legs.

Your child may also be sensitive to certain sounds, and you can find ways to desensitize him. For example, you can record the sound of a fire alarm and allow your child to listen to it repeatedly, gradually letting the volume rise as he goes.

Visual overload. You child can actually experience a visual overload, making him feel that there is just too many things aiming for his eyes. It can be overwhelming for his brain to process all the things around him, such as too many people that are constantly moving and ceiling fans that are swirling on top of his head, which make it difficult for him to focus. Your child may also find it bothersome and visually distracting to have fluorescent lights around him, especially since his hypersensitive eyes can actually detect any flicker.

Help your child manage visual overload by avoiding the use of fluorescent lights altogether. If this is not possible, you can transfer his desk to a place near a window, or you can replace the fluorescent light with new bulbs, which do not flicker as much. You can also keep the flickering of fluorescent lights to a minimum by placing next to your child's desk a lamp fitted with an incandescent bulb.

Eating issues. It can be hard for your child with autism to deal with lunch times, especially if he is still in nursery school. He might be hypersensitive to particular flavors or textures of food. He may also have this fear of tasting unfamiliar foods. You may also find it difficult to have your child sit down at a table and eat since he is overactive.

What is important is that you see progress in your child as you help him deal with his eating issues. As eating with other children can be an overwhelming situation for your child, you may try letting him eat on his own at first, and then gradually invite other children over at his table.

It also helps to make your child follow a strictly consistent lunchtime routine. You can take out a table mat as a cue that it's time for him to sit at the table to eat. Make sure that your child eats only when he is sitting down. If he stands up and moves around, encourage him to always go back to his chair, sit down, and eat, even for just a couple of minutes.

Toileting dilemmas. Toileting dilemmas are common in some children with autism. Because he has no idea of what is appropriate, your child may do his toileting in different places besides the toilet. It helps to create a toilet routine for your child to follow. After his meal, wait for twenty minutes, and then can encourage your child to go to the toilet.

Toy problems. The act of choosing what toy to play with or what game to have fun with can be a difficult task for a child with autism. Instead of choosing a toy, your child may stand in a corner and become engaged in flicking his fingers or another activity that is self-stimulatory. It helps to gradually introduce choices to your child so that he is not too overwhelmed. You could try offering a new toy that he could use in his favorite playtime activity.

Playtime can also be challenging to your child as he may have not yet developed his skills in self-occupancy, as well as the imagination needed for him to scrutinize and experiment with his toys. You can let your child play with functional toys, which are not necessarily things he has to play with, but will allow him to have something appropriate and constructive to occupy himself with.

It also helps to have these toys around as much as possible, as becoming familiar with them can encourage him to use them more often. This in turn helps your child develop his ability to choose a toy or game.

Socialization concerns. Helping your child socialize is the best thing you can do for him. Although he may appear to dislike playing with other children, it is not because he does not want to. The reason may simply be his inability or lack of knowledge on how to join a game or strike up a conversation. You can teach your child the ways in which he can enjoy playing with other kids. You may also encourage other children to invite him to join them in their game.

It helps to keep in mind that your child does best in play activities that are structured, ones that have a definite start and end. Coach your child on reading other people's emotions, body language, and facial expressions. He may end up laughing at others because he simply does not know how to react or what to say; you can teach him to ask other children how they are feeling.

Chapter 5 Ensuring Your Child's Happiness

Understandably, what worries you most as a parent of a child with autism is the fact that the time will come when you are no longer around to be there for him and to take care of his needs. To ensure that your child has a shot at having a happy life when you are gone, consider the following tips:

On His Own

Equip your child with social skills. The most crucial thing you can teach your child while ensuring that he lives a happy life is social skills (some ideas were given in the previous chapter). Admittedly, helping your child overcome his problem behaviors or develop good communication skills is as important as teaching him social skills.

But it helps to think of how your child fares in the long run, especially when he reaches the age of forty. By that time, you can count on a great number of people, including health care providers, to be willing to be with him, regardless of the fact that he does not talk much and may be inclined to hit them.

What is important is that your child develops the ability to connect with other people, who are more than likely to adore his pleasant personality, engaging smile, or earnest hug. It also helps to remember that when your child learns how to reach out to and surround himself with other people, he is less likely to get lonely, and therefore more likely to be happy.

It will be in your child's best interest to focus your time and energy on teaching him to socialize with other people. There are a lot of books and videos you can gather information from on how to uncover the lovable person inside your child's body.

Create a happy-future plan for your child. Your child can hardly eat well on his own, so it is essential that you establish a plan that ensures he has happiness in the future. Aside from preparing necessities like letters of intent and special needs trusts for your child, you cannot go wrong with having a life quality plan in place for him. Make sure that all areas of his life are covered in the plan, such as residential requirements, friendships opportunities, and recreational needs.

Encourage your child to have passionate interests. Your child will be more likely to be happy in life if he engages in things that he has a passionate interest in. In fact, the more interests he has, the better. Children and adults who have autism often have interests that could even provide them a career in the future.

Help your child develop and nurture these interests. When has many things to occupy himself with, the more happy and at ease he feels with himself, and the easier it is for people to be around him. Provide your child plenty of opportunities to engage in his passionate interests. Make sure that all the people around him know about them.

Take steps to make your child a valuable member of society. Contrary to what most people believe, you can help your child make valuable contributions to society. It does not even have anything to do with cleaning tables or recycling. Your child can become a valuable friend to a person living in a nursing home, or he can do community volunteering (such as painting the houses of poor people in the neighborhood) every month with other group members.

He can also be a member of certain organization (church, homeowners, business owners, art class, or reading club). The important thing is that your child builds connections to the people around him.

Enlist the assistance of caring people. It would do your child a world of good if you ensure that there will be people (excluding paid staff or health care providers) around to help him when you are gone. You can start your own support group (it can be formal or otherwise) consisting of people who have autistic family members. This way, you have people who are sure to take up where you left off.

In The Meantime

But while you are still present, here are things you can do to ensure your child's happiness:

Trust your gut feeling. It helps to go the extra mile for your child. You most probably have this feeling that somewhere deep within your child's body is a child who thinks and feels. Although the hidden gifts of your child are buried down by all the confusion as well as challenges that his condition comes with, rest assured that your child is "there." You cannot box your child within his problematic behaviors or confusing quirks.

By working patiently, deliberately, and lovingly with your child, you can most certainly overcome all the hurdles of autism. You do not even have to take a shot at achieving some semblance of normalcy. Know that your child is capable of great things when you focus on his strengths instead of dwelling on and trying to repair his vulnerabilities.

Enter your child's world. Nothing beats in joining your child in his world when it comes to ensuring his happiness. By joining him, you get to know the reasons behind his problematic behaviors, which are usually signs that not everything is alright, whether inside or outside their bodies.

No matter how long it may take you, try breaking down the messages behind your child's actions, and then communicate to him in ways that he will be able to understand. Your child will benefit from your teaching him the nitty-gritty of ordinary things without any hint of judgment. This makes him feel that he can safely learn from you and lead him to thrive better.

Broaden your child's world. It is not enough to enter your child's world. You also have to look for ways in which you can broaden it, which is the only way for him to gain more experience and understand things better. You can allow him to engage in physical tasks. Encourage him to try some activities, which might be unfamiliar to him at first, so that he will be able to feel his body moving in space.

You can also encourage your child to develop his interests into skills that he can use to communicate with and connect to others. Let him grow out of his comfort zone and unleash his creativity, and then let him know that you appreciate him for it.

Love your child without ifs or buts. Unconditional love is something that everybody needs, but it is absolutely essential to your child's well-being and happiness. Never let him hear you say or make him feel like "if only you could…" or "why is it so hard for you to…?"

Your child can feel things, even if he is unable to express it. He does not need to feel that you have expectations that he has not lived up to. Your child did not choose to be born with autism – he never asked to be born in this world, period. You owe it to him to love, guide, and support him in his journey with autism.

Practice plenty of patience. You need a huge dose of patience on a daily basis to be able to help your child have a happy life despite his condition. It helps to start thinking of his autism as a unique ability and stop viewing it as some form of disability. Acknowledge his limitations but do not dwell on them and focus on his strengths instead.

For example, your child may not be good at making conversation or even just a simple eye contact, but he surely should be praised for not lying to anyone, cheating at games, or judging other people. Finally, you can obtain much patience from the mere fact that your child solely relies on you to be his foundation, guide, and advocate. Don't let him down.

Recognize your child's meltdown triggers. Your child can experience meltdowns, and it is important that you know what triggers them. You may feel horrible whenever your child acts up, but the experience is actually more horrible for him. The reason for his meltdown could be overloading of his senses, or being pushed past his abilities in social situations.

Consider recording your child's meltdown times, settings, as well as the people involved or around. You might be surprised to notice a pattern, such as he may act up when he does not know what is happening around him so that he does not know how to react; he may have trouble getting to sleep; or he may be having gastrointestinal problems or food allergies. It is up to you to detect signs of distress (emotional, mental, or physical) in your child, as he is unable to tell you that he is having them.

CHAPTER 6: Guidelines for Parents to Help a Child with Autism at home

If you have as of late discovered that your youngster has or may have a mental imbalance range issue, you're most likely pondering and agonizing over what comes next. No guardian is ever arranged to hear that a youngster is something besides glad and solid, and an analysis of Autism can be especially terrifying. You may be uncertain about how to best help your tyke or confounded by clashing treatment guidance. On the other hand you may have been informed that Autism is a hopeless, long lasting condition, abandoning you worried that nothing you do will have any kind of effect.

While beyond any doubt a mental imbalance is not something an individual essentially "develops out of," there are numerous medicines that can help youngsters learn new aptitudes and conquer a wide mixture of formative difficulties. From free taxpayer supported organizations to in-home behavioral treatment and school-based projects, help is accessible to meet your youngster's unique needs. With the right treatment arrangement, and a ton of adoration and backing, your tyke can learn, develop, and flourish.

Guideline for Parents: Things You Have to Do to Support Your Child

As the guardian of a kid with a mental imbalance or related formative defers, the best thing you can do is to begin treatment immediately. Look for help when you think something's incorrectly. Try not to hold up to check whether your kid will look up some other time or exceed the issue. Try not to try and sit tight for an official finding. The prior youngsters with autism range issue get help, the more noteworthy their shot of treatment achievement. Early intercession is the best approach to accelerate your kid's improvement and diminish the manifestations of a mental imbalance.

- **Learn More About Autism Disorder:** The more you think about a mental imbalance range issue, the better prepared you'll be to settle on educated choices for your tyke. Teach yourself about the treatment choices, make inquiries, and take part in all treatment choices.

- **Become a Specialist:** Make sense of what triggers your child's "awful" or problematic practices and what inspires a positive reaction. What does your mentally unbalanced kid find unpleasant? Cooling? Uncomfortable? Agreeable? In the event that you comprehend what influences your tyke, you'll be better at investigating issues and anticipating circumstances that cause challenges.

- **Accept Your Child:** As opposed to concentrating on how your mentally unbalanced kid is unique in relation to other kids and what he or she is "missing," practice acknowledgement. Appreciate your child's exceptional idiosyncrasies, praise little triumphs, and quit contrasting your kid with others. Feeling unequivocally cherished and acknowledged will help your tyke more than whatever else.

- **Try not to Give Up:** It is difficult to foresee the course of a mental imbalance range issue. Try not to make a hasty judgment about what life will be similar to for your kid. Like others, individuals with a mental imbalance have a whole lifetime to develop and build up their capacities.

Tips One for Parents: Create a Safety Zone for Your Child

Gather as much knowledge as you can about Autism and getting included in treatment will go far toward helping your tyke. Also, the accompanying tips will make every day home life simpler for both you and your extremely introverted kid:

Be Steady: Kids with a mental imbalance have some major snags adjusting what they've realized in one setting, (for example, the specialist's office or school) to others, including the home. Case in point, your youngster may utilize gesture based communication at school to convey, however never think to do as such at home. Making consistency in your kid's surroundings is the most ideal approach to strengthen learning. Discover what your tyke's advisors are doing and proceed with their strategies at home. Investigate the likelihood of having treatment occur in more than one spot to urge your tyke to exchange what he or she has gained starting with one environment then onto the next. It's additionally critical to be predictable in the way you associate with your tyke and manage testing practices.

Stick to a Timetable: Youngsters with a mental imbalance have a tendency to do best when they have a profoundly organized calendar or schedule. Once more, this backtracks to the consistency they both need and hunger for. Set up a timetable for your tyke, with consistent times for suppers, treatment, school, and sleep time.

Attempt to keep interruptions to this routine to a base. On the off chance that there is an unavoidable timetable change, set up your kid for it ahead of time.

Compensate Good Behavior: Uplifting feedback can run far with youngsters with autism, so attempt to "find them doing something great." Praise them when they act suitably or take in another ability, being certain about what conduct they're being adulated for. Likewise search for different approaches to compensate them for good conduct, for example, issuing them a sticker or giving them a chance to play with a most loved toy.

Make a Home-safety Zone: Cut out a private space in your home where your youngster can unwind, feel secure, and be safe. This will include arranging and defining limits in ways your kid can get it. Visual signs can be useful. You might likewise need to security proof the house, especially if your kid is inclined to fits of rage or other self-harmful practices.

Tips Two for Parents: Learn Nonverbal Way of Communication

Associating with a tyke with Autism can be testing, yet you don't have to talk so as to impart and bond. You impart by the way you take a gander at your tyke, the way you touch him or her, and by the tone of your voice and your non-verbal communication. Your youngster is additionally speaking with you, regardless of the possibility that he or she never talks. You simply need to take in the dialect.

Search for Nonverbal Signs: In the event that you are perceptive and mindful, you can figure out how to get on the nonverbal signals that youngsters with autism utilization to convey. Pay consideration on the sorts of sounds they make, their outward appearances, and the motions they utilize when they're drained, hungry, or need something.

Try to Understand the Needs of Your Child: It is just characteristic to feel upset when you are misconstrued or overlooked, and it is the same for youngsters with autism. At the point when kids with a mental imbalance showcase, it is regularly in light of the fact that you're not getting on their nonverbal signs. Having a fit is their direction conveying their disappointment and standing out enough to be noticed.

Arrange Time for Fun: A youngster adapting to autism is still a child. For both kids with autism and their guardians, there necessities to be more to life than treatment. Plan recess when your youngster is most ready and conscious. Make sense of approaches to have a fabulous time together by contemplating the things that make your youngster grin, chuckle, and leave their shell. Your youngster is liable to appreciate these exercises most in the event that they don't appear to be remedial or instructive. There are gigantic advantages that outcome from your delight in your kid's organization and from your tyke's satisfaction in investing unpressurized energy with you. Have a crucial impact of learning and shouldn't feel like work.

Pay Attention on the Sensitiveness of Your Child: Numerous youngsters with a mental imbalance are touchy to light, solid, touch, taste, and smell. Other kids with a mental imbalance are "under-touchy" to tangible boosts. Make sense of what sights, sounds, scents, developments, and material sensations trigger your child's "terrible" or troublesome practices and what inspires a positive reaction. What does your extremely introverted tyke find distressing? Cooling? Uncomfortable? Pleasant? On the off chance that you comprehend what influences your kid, you'll be better at investigating issues, anticipating circumstances that cause challenges, and making effective encounters.

Tips Three for Parents: Create a Personal Treatment Plan for Your Child

With such a large number of diverse a mental imbalance medicines accessible, and it can be hard to make sense of which approach is ideal for your youngster. Making things more confused, you may hear diverse or notwithstanding clashing suggestions from folks and specialists. At the point when assembling an autism treatment arrangement for your youngster, remember that there is no single treatment that will work for everybody. Every individual on a mental imbalance range is novel, with distinctive qualities and shortcomings. Your youngster's treatment ought to be customized by or her individual needs. You know your tyke best, so its dependent upon you to verify those needs are being met.

Remember that regardless of what a mental imbalance treatment arrangement is picked, your inclusion is essential to achievement. You can help your tyke get the most out of treatment by meeting expectations as one with the autism treatment group and finishing the treatment at home.

Concerning a mental imbalance treatment, there are a confounding mixture of treatments and methodologies. Some a mental imbalance treatments concentrate on lessening tricky practices and building correspondence and social abilities, while others manage tactile mix issues, engine aptitudes, intense subject matters, and nourishment sensitivities.

With such a large number of decisions, it is amazingly critical to do your examination, converse with a mental imbalance treatment specialists, and make inquiries. At the same time, remember that you don't need to pick only one sort of treatment. The objective of autism treatment ought to be to treat the majority of your kid's side effects and needs. This frequently obliges a joined treatment approach that exploits a wide range of sorts of treatment.

Regular autism medicines incorporate conduct treatment, discourse dialect treatment, play-based treatment, active recuperation, word related treatment, and nutritious treatment.

Tips Four for Parents: Find Support and Help for Your Child

Caring for Autistic can request a ton of vitality and time. There may be days when you feel overpowered, focused on, or demoralized. Child rearing isn't ever simple, and bringing up a youngster with exceptional needs is significantly additionally difficult. So as to be the best parent you can be, it is key that you deal with yourself. Try not to attempt to do everything all alone. You don't need to! There are numerous spots that groups of extremely introverted children can swing to for guidance, some assistance, support and advocacy:

Autism Care Groups: Joining a mental imbalance care group is an extraordinary approach to meet different families managing the same difficulties you are. Folks can impart data, get counsel, and incline toward one another for enthusiastic backing. Simply being around others in almost the same situation and imparting their experience can go far toward diminishing the seclusion numerous folks feel in the wake of getting a tyke's a mental imbalance determination.

Break Care: Every guardian needs a break every so often. Also, for folks adapting to the included anxiety of a mental imbalance, this is particularly genuine. In rest consideration, another guardian assumes control briefly, showing you a bit of mercy for a couple of hours, days, or even weeks. To discover break care alternatives in your general vicinity.

Individual, Conjugal, or Family Guiding: If anxiety, tension, or sorrow is getting to you, you may need to see your very own specialist. Treatment is a sheltered spot where you can speak sincerely about all that you're feeling—the great, the terrible, and the appalling. Marriage or family treatment can likewise bail you work out issues that the difficulties of existence with a mentally unbalanced tyke are creating in your spousal relationship.

Conclusion

I hope this book is able to help you to realize that having a child with autism does not have to make you feel too overwhelmed to face a life with your child that is full of challenges.

Loving and enjoying your child for who he is, is the key to effectively managing his condition as well as allowing him to grow to be a happy child.

The next step is to find ways on becoming your own child's expert in all matters regarding autism. Aim to be the best solutions provider whenever your child finds himself in uncomfortable or difficult situations. And never forget to take care of yourself in the process of looking after your child's needs, as your child will lose any chances of being happy if you are not comfortable or stress-free yourself. Know that your well-being is more essential to your child's life than any professional treatment.